**The Not Perfect but Better Diet**
**Riverhouse Publishing**
**St. Louis MO 63146**
**ISBN: 1-893892-02-6**

© **1998, 2007, 2010 Cris Robins**

# Dedication

This work is dedicated to all the people who try every day
to be better than they were the day before;
who try to be their best;
and to G-d, who knows this most of all …
we are not perfect,
just striving to be better.

## About the Cover

Some would question as to why I would put a photo of a tree on the cover of a diet book. The simple answer is this – why not? Yes, I know most diet books have pictures of fabulous looking people who are in great shape gracing their covers; however, this is about being NOT PERFECT, so why would I show a picture of someone … perfect?

This tree is very special to me; what you can't see is the mobile home that sat behind it and the house that sat in front of it; the first being where I raised my children for about 18 years, the second where my in-laws (in blessed memory) raised their eight children and many grandchildren. The reason you can't see these things is not because I took them out of the picture, but because when my mother-in-law passed on, the farmer who had bought the 26 acres, bulldozed down all the buildings.

I thought something should be left in memory of them.

# About the author

My name is Cris Robins; I am a writer by trade and talent. I researched this diet because I needed one; I use this diet because it works for me. Some of my friends and family have used it to with mixed results; the mix comes in when they chose not to do it.

I wish you well.

# Table of Contents

# In the beginning …

In January 1998 I went in for a routine checkup where after a couple of tests were run I found out my cholesterol was 233 and my weight was 206 pounds. (That may not sound bad if you AREN'T a woman who only stands 5'7.) My 300+ pound doctor scared the daylights out of me by saying I was a walking heart attack. When you've not yet hit forty, those are frightening words. So, I did what I always do when I'm frightened … I quit eating. After a week I wised up and did what I should have done in the first place … went back to see my regular doctor.

He was an old doctor and not much worried him. Together we sat down and tackled the problem; he told me what I couldn't eat, I figured out what I could in accord with the health guidelines. By July I'd went from 206 to 176 and my cholesterol dropped to 185. But, we discovered another problem; I was staring diabetes in the face. My Triglycerides were 269 when they should have ranged between 120 and 150. After 20 minutes of going through every single food that could possibly be causing this high of a sugar intake (the usual cookies, ice cream, soda routine) he hit upon coffee. Of course I drink coffee, somewhere between 12 and 20 cups a day; with three teaspoons of sugar and two teaspoons of creamer in each one. This totaled about 15 POUNDS of sugar a month.

He recommended I go on a diabetic diet. The problem was, I

found out, there isn't one. There are also no guidelines for the amount of sugar one should consume on a daily basis. So, I asked the American Diabetes Association if I limited my consumption to one teaspoonful a day if this would be a good guide. When the woman finished laughing, she said, "Good luck."

Well, how many grams of sugar are in one teaspoon? I don't mean a measuring teaspoon, because who really measures the sugar for their coffee with one of them? So, I asked my brother the scientist to take one teaspoon of sugar and measure it: 11 to 14 grams, depending on whether it's heaped or not. So, there's the guide. I switched from sugar to fake sweetener for my coffee, made a couple of other minor changes, and went from 176 to 136 by December and my Triglycerides dropped to 119.

But, I had gone TOO FAR. My mother burst out crying when she saw the "new me" as she was certain I had cancer. My doctor about had a nervous breakdown and warned if I hit 130 pounds that I was going to be in the hospital. So my doctor and I agreed on what I SHOULD weigh; 140-145. Although it was kind of fun putting on the four pounds like everything else, I learned all things in moderation; I still should have asked him FIRST what I should weigh before I just started losing weight; as you should ask yours first as well. Am I still on the diet several years later? Yes, I am. My cholesterol is about 185; Triglycerides are 119; and my weight is 144; a very solid size eight. ☺

Here's to being, not perfect, but better.

# Step One

You've been there -- let's face it -- we all have. We've been 5, 10, 15, 20, 50 (or more!) pounds over weight. So we go on a crash diet; crash and burn that is; and end up gaining more than what we lost; until now.

It's difficult to know who to believe. Every time you turn on the television or radio or open a newspaper there's a new scientific study to show eggs and pork and wheat bran are all the rage; only to have another study contradict it. Who to believe? Where to turn? Here is the truth:

~~ No one really knows. ~~

The only thing anyone knows for certain is we must eat. To this end the American Cancer Society, the American Heart Association, and the Federal Department of Agricultural (FDA) have issued their guidelines telling us how much and of what we are to eat. They don't, however, tell us how to cook the food to get the best nutritional value from it or how to eliminate the fat from our bodies.

It takes about two ounces of common sense to figure out what goes in our mouths contributes to our overall health. As the fad of the day is fat is out, I've taken the guides from the above and designed a diet to limit the amount of fat we intake. Thus, the less fat we eat; the less we have to lose! :)

But this is more than just a diet, it's a lifestyle. I challenge you to make meals fun, light, delicious and suitable for the whole family. Some of the areas I cover include the following:

The difference between fat and cholesterol

How to cut the fat and increase the flavor

Real foods for real people -- menus for everyday

How to eat at a fast food joint without going off your diet!

The idea behind step one of this diet is to lower cholesterol levels and lose weight. (Step Two is to lower sugar.) The guidelines for good health (from the above sources) are 200 mg of cholesterol a day with 64 grams of fat; we're looking for 0 mg of cholesterol and 20 mg of fat. After all, this is designed to be a low fat -- no cholesterol diet. Studies show humans do not need cholesterol, but they do need fat.

So what's the difference? The difference comes in what you eat. Fat, when eaten, makes the body's own cholesterol, in addition it is responsible for getting oxygen to the heart and lungs. Very useful indeed!

Cholesterol, when eaten, however is responsible for clogging the arteries -- not a pretty picture; and not much else.

Confused? You're not alone.

Cholesterol is an animal bi-product and is found in meats, milk, butter, cheese, other dairy products and some nuts. You can't really SEE cholesterol. Fat is found in all of the above also -- however, you can see it. It's that slimy little piece of nothing on your meat, chicken and other foods.

We've all heard of the good and bad cholesterol -- HDL being good and LDL being bad. In a nut shell: HDL cleans cholesterol out of the body's system; LDL clogs the arteries. When your intake of cholesterol lowers, so is the need for the good cholesterol. When your intake of fat increases weight gain occurs.

With all of this said, you can see why you need to cut the cholesterol and monitor the fat.

## The Diet

So here's the DO NOT EAT list: bacon and sausage. (Short, eh?)

Eat, but in moderation: eggs and salad dressings.

Eat all you want: any fresh fruits, vegetables, grains, and pastas.

An added bonus: to help your body lower your current cholesterol faster, every morning with your coffee, eat two fiber wafers; cholesterol has a habit of clinging to fiber and when the fiber is "eliminated" some of the cholesterol goes with it.

# Substitutions

| For | Substitute |
| --- | --- |
| Butter | No fat butter – but not margarine. |
| Oil/butter (in recipes) | Applesauce for baked goods, Canola oil for salads. |
| Vit. D Milk | 2% milk (skim if you can stand it.) |
| Cooking oil | Cooking spray -- or for sautéing, water. |
| Mayo | Salad dressing or sandwich spread (really low in cholesterol!) Fat free if you can stand it. |
| Salad dressings | Fat free dressing in variety of flavors. |
| Sour Cream | Fat free is wonderful and real is a nice treat. |
| Chip dip | Fat free is a bit salty but good. |
| Eggs | For both cooking and baking, fake eggs (brand of your choice) works well. Fake eggs are considered egg products that are made using only the egg whites and not the yolks. I use the term "fake eggs" because |

| | |
|---|---|
| | "egg product" doesn't sound like something I'd want to eat. |
| Cheeses | Low fat, no cholesterol, but they can be a bit pricey. |
| Bacon | Fat free bacon bits. (I don't care for the frozen type of bacon.) |
| Sausage | Sorry, nothing. Just quit eating it. Even turkey sausage is high in fat. |
| Noodles | Noodles derive their fat from eggs; so, noodles made without the yolk of the egg is the better choice. |

## At the grocery store

Read before you buy. Now the first couple of times, this is going to be a pain. Pick up EVERY SINGLE item and read the label. If it is low in fat and a big zero in cholesterol it goes in the cart. If it is under 10 mg cholesterol a few go in. Unless it is meat or chicken it should NOT be over 20 mg of cholesterol per serving. (Most of this can be eliminated in the cooking process.) Look for skinless/boneless chicken and hamburger in the 90% fat free category. Do not by-pass pork! Believe it or not, some pork is actually lower than chicken. Trimming the visible fat (or boiling first) really helps here. Be aware of turkey products. They are not always the best choice.

Many foods have hidden fat/cholesterol levels. Some include: cookies, crackers, cereal (yeah, I know!), non-dairy coffee creamer, salad dressings, chocolate, bottled or canned anything, frozen or quick foods; turkey products and lunchmeats.

## Cooking tips

It doesn't make dieting easier if you take a skinless/boneless chicken breast and deep fry it in oil or bake it in butter. Cooking is the key to this diet. It is not difficult and sometimes can be easier with less clean up then how you cook now.

If you are going to deep fry something use Canola oil (if you can stand the taste) or Wesson's vegetable oil (it's not quite as high as the others). After the food is cooked, dab with a paper towel to remove the excessive oil. (I do this in restaurants when I order a hamburger and the looks are fun to watch!)

Meats have their own fat. You don't need to put oil in a pan to fry a hamburger! This just doubles the fat content. Instead, heat the pan, put the meat in (it should sizzle), brown on both sides, then cover for a few minutes. While the meat is cooking, its own fat will coat the pan so it won't stick. Remove the lid about half way through the cooking time. This system will work with every type of meat, including chicken. One note:

before cooking the meat, trim all visible signs of fat from the meat/chicken. This just cut the cholesterol by almost half. Try to microwave meat ONLY when you have to. I've found using the microwave, even to defrost, has a tendency to dry out the meat, make it tough or give it a funny taste.

Using a gas grill or electric one works very well for getting out the fat -- but has its drawbacks. If you can afford it, (as it costs up to $100!) there are many new grills/frying pans on the market which will cut the fat and cooking time.

Vegetables: Microwave or steam all veggies. (Unless you prefer them raw.) Do not use butter! After the veggies are cooked use the Fleishmann's to season. No fat and it tastes good. They even have a no fat cheese topping, too. For baked potatoes, use the no fat sour cream or better yet, use salsa. (Ummmm. Good stuff!)

Carbs, i.e. pasta, rice, noodles: Here is where you really have to be careful. Although most pastas and rices have no fat or cholesterol of their own, the sauces are normally full of it! Noodles, of course, are usually made with eggs. However, the noodles made without the egg yolks are the best.

To flavor carbs, before cooking add about a teaspoon of chicken bouillon granules to the water and eliminate the salt called for in your recipe. After cooking, use either the butter substitute or veggies sauces. (I prefer the vegetable sauce.) I've got a really good rice recipe which adds black-eyed peas and salsa -- wonderful stuff. (And can be found on the back of the rice box.)

Speaking of salsa -- it's the diet sauce of choice. To flavor anything from soup to chicken, use salsa ... no fat, no cholesterol.

# Look before you eat!

As you sit to the table, look at your plate. Determine which of the foods is the highest in fat/cholesterol. Eat that last! Start with the salad, the carbs, then the meat. Is there one of each food group? This is tricky ... if you are having a casserole; do you have meat, carbs, veggies and dairy in there? If not, could you alter it to? Think about it.

Break down each of the items on your plate to their lowest form. A bowl of cereal with vitamin D milk and fruit has about 60 mg of cholesterol; where the same bowl with 2% milk has about 25 mg (and if you only put on 1/2 cup of milk it's down to 12.5 mg!).

Look at each of the salad components: lettuce, tomato, carrots, cucumbers, peppers, onions, mushrooms; all good so far. But did you add: cheese, bacon, croutons, or Ranch dressing? This can be as high as a steak sandwich.

# Real meals, for real people

## Breakfast ideas

| | |
|---|---|
| Cereal | Any type with zero cholesterol and no or little fat. |
| Milk for above | 2% or skim -- 1/2 cup preferred. |
| Fruit | Applesauce, bananas, strawberries, etc. |
| Juice | Pineapple, apple, tomato, orange, etc. |

Total:   20 mg of cholesterol -- as low as 12.5 if you use 1/2 cup and zero if you use skim milk. (Note:  Compare the above to a balanced diet: grains, dairy and two fruit/veggie sources ... not bad at all.)

---

| | |
|---|---|
| Scrambled eggs | Fake eggs |
| Toast (no cholesterol bread) | With butter substitute |
| Fruit | Applesauce, bananas, strawberries, etc. |
| Juice | Pineapple, apple, tomato, orange, etc. |

Total:  About zero cholesterol.

--

| | |
|---|---|
| French toast | Fake eggs and bread |
| Fruit | Applesauce, bananas, strawberries, etc. |
| Juice | Pineapple, apple, tomato, orange, etc. |

Total: About zero cholesterol.

---

All out breakfast!

| | |
|---|---|
| Scrambled eggs | Fake eggs |
| Hashbrowns | Fried with cooking spray and adding peppers and onions. |
| Bacon | No fat variety |
| Toast | With butter substitute |
| Fruit | Applesauce, bananas, strawberries, etc. |
| Juice | Pineapple, apple, tomato, orange, etc. |

Grand total:  About 10 mg of cholesterol!! Cut the bacon and you've got about zero.

# Lunch

Ham or turkey sandwich
(two slices meat)

Using no cholesterol bread, Miracle Whip
dressing and turkey based lunchmeat.
Top with onion, tomato and lettuce for an
an added serving of veggies bonus!

Salad — Veggies of choice and fat free dressing.

Juice, diet soda, water — Try to throw in a fruit juice here.

Total:  25 mg of cholesterol and about 5 grams of fat. Use mustard
instead of dressing and deduct 5 mg of cholesterol and 1 gram of fat.

---

Peanut butter sandwich — No cholesterol bread and peanut butter.

Jam — Can also use apple butter.

Soup — Watch the cans on this one. They may say

zero fat/

cholesterol -- but then you need to add milk
to make them.

Juice — Just for balance.

Total:  zero cholesterol, about 16 mg of fat.

---

Pasta salad

Be careful here due to the bacon bits and
salad dressing. Substitute the mayo for fat
free ranch dressing for a change. Add a can
of peas or mixed veggies to boost the
balanced diet.

Fruit — Any of your choice.

Total:  zero, again

----

# The last meal of the day

Here is where most of the fat comes into play -- and just before bedtime, no less.

The basic diet is: lean meat/chicken, carbs, veggies and/or fruit.

- Meat should be grilled, baked, fried in its own fat, or boiled/broiled.
- Potatoes should be boiled (add a bit of bouillon or dill) or micro-waved. Fried is not good here as the fat seems to vary from breakfast.
- Noodles or pasta with dried parmesan cheese is a nice change. Rice is always a plus if you don't put eggs in it.
- Salads are always welcomed if they are just veggies and fat free dressing.
- Fruit straight from the can (chilled) is a nice dessert or topping for dinner.
- Cereal straight from the box is the snack of choice.

# A word about portions

If you noticed, I didn't say, the equivalent of two eggs worth of fake eggs, or one apple, or four slices of fake bacon. The key here is not how many servings, but the fat/cholesterol per serving. If there is NO fat or cholesterol in a two-egg serving of fake eggs, there is also NO fat or cholesterol in a four-egg serving. NO means NO.

Now, where you need to be careful is in the fat content, if there is one gram of fat in the fake bacon per two slices, and you eat four slices, then you've eaten two grams of fat. Be aware of the per-serving measurements and eat accordingly.

# Dining out

Being on a diet is a lifestyle change, not a once in a while event. It doesn't mean you need to stop going to the hamburger joint or the corner cafe once in a while.

But just like at home, watch what you eat. Order your burger with everything on the side. Lift the bun, dab the grease off and leave the mayo in the little plastic cup. Ask for salsa, too. Watch the way the food is cooked. Is it broiled chicken or deep fried? Get a baked potato (with butter and sour cream on the side) instead of French fries. If given a choice, go with the sour cream, not the cheese sauce and butter. It makes you feel decadent and is lower in fat!

In the mood for a pizza? Get it with chicken, veggies, salsa and low-fat cheese.

# Important things to remember!

1.	Once you start, you may find it very difficult to go back. This is no joke. After you've cut the fat down and the cholesterol out of your diet, you will get sick from eating food high in both. A pizza with all the trimmings will make you throw up! (I did this just last night, and knew better before I ate it!) Consider yourself warned. Eating a sausage breakfast sandwich with all the trimmings will throw your system into overdrive; complete with nausea, tummy cramps, and gas. (Um, again, the voice of experience!)

2.	Remember to eat enough! You need between 1700 and 2000 calories a day (even when dieting). This may not seem like much, but it is! Try to break the calories up between the three meals. On 1700 it's 565(+-) per meal. On 2000 it's 665 (+-) per meal. If you can't eat that much in one meal, add a fourth meal per day. For example: eat at 6 am, 10 am, 2 pm and 6 pm. Try to keep your last meal about three hours before bedtime; this gives the food time to start digesting and not allowing it all to turn to fat.

3.	This does not mean you can't splurge. Once every two weeks eat something special...chocolate cake comes to mind. (Here's a really nice little trick -- bake the cake yourself! Use applesauce instead of oil; and fake eggs instead of eggs. It's the best of both worlds -- low fat/ cholesterol and great tasting!) Go to a fast food joint. Just be careful.

You will find a million different ways to go off your diet, just do one of them once every two weeks.

4.　　Adjust your current recipes with the substitutions. You'd be surprised at how the taste rarely differs but the cholesterol does.

5.　　Be aware of your friends and family members. Once the weight starts to come off, your friends may become less than friendly. Throw a dinner party inviting them and fix your favorite low fat dishes. They won't believe you eat so well.

Have fun with it! Make it a challenge to find the lowest possible cholesterol level on any one meal.

**Before starting this, or any diet, check with your doctor or health care professional first.** You may want to also ask them what they think your weight should be before you begin.

# Step Two

That is step one, this step two. As I said before, there are no tried and true guidelines for how much sugar one needs on a daily basis. The recommendation is: less than what you're eating now. For me, that doesn't say anything.

So, I settled on one teaspoon a day. Most doctors and health care professionals will not believe you can do this. The first step is seeing what your Triglycerides level is before you begin; the range is 120-150 for most people. It's a simple blood test that most doctors will jump at the chance to give you while they are checking your cholesterol level. Ask them what it should be then you will know what you need to shoot for. The second step is looking at what you are eating to find the sugar demons. Is it the low fat/no cholesterol ice cream? Or maybe those delicious fat free cookies? Is your cereal sabotaging you with no fat but 14 grams of sugar per serving? Or, like with me, is it the coffee loaded with sugar and cream? See, they fit step one, but not step two.

The goal is one teaspoon, or a maximum of 14 grams, of sugar per day. Remember that most listings for sugar is per serving; however, most containers are multi-servings. A perfect example is a can of soda. With a listing of 18.4 grams of sugar per serving, it doesn't sound too bad until you realize the can was 2.5 servings. Some of the newer cans actually list one can as one serving. (Like the one I pulled from my fridge to site as an example.)

Just because it's a bag of cookies, doesn't mean it's a serving. Now, you may be thinking this limits the amount of choices you have when putting together meals. Well, in the above meal plans, the only real sugar comes from the fruit and vegetables. So, keep an eye on the hidden sugars and you should do well.

# A week's worth of real meals, for real people

## Monday

### Breakfast

| | |
|---|---|
| Cereal | Any type with zero cholesterol and no or little fat. |
| Milk for above | 2% or skim -- 1/2 cup preferred. |
| Fruit | Applesauce, bananas, strawberries, etc. |
| Juice | Pineapple, apple, tomato, orange, etc. |

Total: 20 mg of cholesterol -- as low as 12.5 if you use 1/2 cup and zero if you use skim milk.

---

### Lunch

| | |
|---|---|
| Ham or turkey sandwich | Using no cholesterol bread, Miracle Whip (two slices meat) dressing and turkey based lunchmeat. Top with onion, tomato and lettuce for an added serving of veggies bonus! |
| Salad | Veggies of choice and fat free dressing. |
| Juice, diet soda, water | Try to throw in a fruit juice here. |

Total: 25 mg of cholesterol and about 5 grams of fat. Use mustard instead of dressing and deduct 5 mg of cholesterol and 1 gram of fat.

### Dinner

The basic diet is: lean meat/chicken, carbs, veggies and/or fruit.

| | |
|---|---|
| Hamburger patty | Fried as directed or broiled, topped with salsa or mustard. |
| Fries | Baked, not fried, with ketchup. |
| Salad | If you want with light dressing. Or veggie |
| Veggie | Any fresh, frozen, boiled, or micro-waved. |
| Fruit | Fresh fruit if it's in season; a banana or orange if not. |
| Drink: | Water, iced tea (no real sugar), coffee or juice |

Total: Depending on the fat of the hamburger, about 20 grams of fat, with 40 mg cholesterol.

**Tuesday**

**Breakfast**

| | |
|---|---|
| Scrambled eggs | Fake eggs |
| Toast (no cholesterol bread) | With butter substitute |
| Fruit | Applesauce, bananas, strawberries, etc. |
| Juice | Pineapple, apple, tomato, orange, etc. |

Total:  About zero cholesterol.

---

**Lunch**

| | |
|---|---|
| Peanut butter sandwich | No cholesterol bread and peanut butter. |
| Jam | Can also use apple butter. |
| Soup | Watch the cans on this one. They may say zero fat/cholesterol -- but then you need to add milk to make them. |
| Juice | Just for balance. |

Total:  zero cholesterol, about 16 mg of fat.

**Dinner**

The basic diet is: lean meat/chicken, carbs, veggies and/or fruit.

| | |
|---|---|
| Chicken/lean pork | Fried as directed or broiled, topped with salsa or dill. |
| Pasta | Noodles; or the flavored packaged kind. |
| Salad | If you want with light dressing. |
| Veggie | Any fresh, frozen, boiled, or micro-waved. |
| Fruit | Fresh fruit if it's in season; a banana or orange if not. |
| Drink: | Water, iced tea (no real sugar), coffee or juice |

Total: Depending on the fat of the hamburger, about 20 grams of fat, with 40 mg of cholesterol.

## Wednesday

### Breakfast

| | |
|---|---|
| French toast | Fake eggs and bread |
| Fruit | Applesauce, bananas, strawberries, etc. |
| Juice | Pineapple, apple, tomato, orange, etc. |

Total: About zero cholesterol.

---

### Lunch

| | |
|---|---|
| Ham or turkey sandwich (two slices meat) | Using no cholesterol bread, Miracle Whip dressing and turkey based lunchmeat. Top with onion, tomato and lettuce for an an added serving of veggies bonus! |
| Salad | Veggies of choice and fat free dressing. |
| Juice, diet soda, water | Try to throw in a fruit juice here. |

Total:  25 mg of cholesterol and about 5 grams of fat. Use mustard instead of dressing and deduct 5 mg of cholesterol and 1 gram of fat.

### Dinner

The basic diet is: lean meat/chicken, carbs, veggies and/or fruit. As it's the middle of the week, you may want to try something fun; meatloaf and mashed potatoes, or a casserole, or grilled meat with grilled veggies. There's nothing wrong with making this an ethnic night either, i.e. Italian (spaghetti and meatballs); Mexican (refried beans, a burrito, or a taco salad); Chinese (sweet and sour chicken with fried rice) or even a night of trying a new recipe; there are tons of them free on line. Have fun with it and get out of your typical box. After all, it's ONLY one meal and it's not going to hurt to try something different. ☺

## Thursday

### Breakfast

| | |
|---|---|
| Cereal | Any type with zero cholesterol and no or little fat. |
| Milk for above | 2% or skim -- 1/2 cup preferred. |
| Fruit | Applesauce, bananas, strawberries, etc. |
| Juice | Pineapple, apple, tomato, orange, etc. |

Total:  20 mg of cholesterol -- as low as 12.5 if you use 1/2 cup and zero if you use skim milk.

---

### Lunch

| | |
|---|---|
| Peanut butter sandwich | No cholesterol bread and peanut butter. |
| Jam | Can also use apple butter. |
| Soup | Watch the cans on this one. They may say zero fat/ cholesterol -- but then you need to add milk to make them. |
| Juice | Just for balance. |

Total:  zero cholesterol, about 16 mg of fat.

### Dinner

The basic diet is: lean meat/chicken, carbs, veggies and/or fruit.

| | |
|---|---|
| Hamburger patty | Fried as directed or broiled, topped with salsa or mustard. |
| Fries | Baked, not fired, with ketchup. |
| Salad | If you want with light dressing. |
| Veggie | Any fresh, frozen, boiled, or micro-waved. |
| Fruit | Fresh fruit if it's in season; a banana or orange if not. |
| Drink: | Water, iced tea (no real sugar), coffee or juice |

Total: Depending on the fat of the hamburger, about 20 grams of fat, with 40 mg of cholesterol.

## Friday

### Breakfast

| | |
|---|---|
| Scrambled eggs | Fake eggs |
| Toast (no cholesterol bread) | With butter substitute |
| Fruit | Applesauce, bananas, strawberries, etc. |
| Juice | Pineapple, apple, tomato, orange, etc. |

Total: About zero cholesterol.

### Lunch

| | |
|---|---|
| Ham or turkey sandwich (two slices meat) | Using no cholesterol bread, Miracle Whip dressing and turkey based lunchmeat. Top with onion, tomato and lettuce for an an added serving of veggies bonus! |
| Salad | Veggies of choice and fat free dressing. |
| Juice, diet soda, water | Try to throw in a fruit juice here. |

Total:  25 mg of cholesterol and about 5 grams of fat. Use mustard instead of dressing and deduct 5 mg of cholesterol and 1 gram of fat.

### Dinner

The basic diet is: lean meat/chicken, carbs, veggies and/or fruit.

| | |
|---|---|
| Chicken/lean pork | Fried as directed or broiled, topped with salsa or dill. |
| Pasta | Noodles; or the flavored packaged kind. |
| Salad | If you want with light dressing. |
| Veggie | Any fresh, frozen, boiled, or micro-waved. |
| Fruit | Fresh fruit if it's in season; a banana or orange if not. |
| Drink: | Water, iced tea (no real sugar), coffee or juice |

Total: Depending on the fat of the hamburger, about 20 grams of fat, with 40 mg of cholesterol.

## Saturday

## Breakfast
All out breakfast!

| | |
|---|---|
| Scrambled eggs | Fake eggs |
| Hashbrowns | Fried with cooking spray and adding peppers and onions. |
| Bacon | No fat variety |
| Toast | With butter substitute |
| Fruit | Applesauce, bananas, strawberries, etc. |
| Juice | Pineapple, apple, tomato, orange, etc. |

Grand total:  About 10 mg of cholesterol!! Cut the bacon and you've got about zero.

## Lunch

| | |
|---|---|
| Pasta salad | Be careful here due to the bacon bits and salad dressing. Substitute the mayo for fat free ranch dressing for a change. Add a can of peas or mixed veggies to boost the balanced diet. |
| Fruit | Any of your choice. |

Total:  zero, again

## Dinner
The basic diet is: lean meat/chicken, carbs, veggies and/or fruit. However, as this is Saturday – splurge and go out for dinner; just be careful to look at your plate so you don't put a week's worth of effort down the drain with a pizza. ☺

## Sunday

### Breakfast
All out breakfast!

| | |
|---|---|
| Scrambled eggs | Fake eggs |
| Hashbrowns | Fried with cooking spray and adding peppers and onions. |
| Bacon | No fat variety |
| Toast | With butter substitute |
| Fruit | Applesauce, bananas, strawberries, etc. |
| Juice | Pineapple, apple, tomato, orange, etc. |

Grand total: About 10 mg of cholesterol!! Cut the bacon and you've got about zero.

### Lunch

| | |
|---|---|
| Pasta salad | Be careful here due to the bacon bits and salad dressing. Substitute the mayo for fat free ranch dressing for a change. Add a can of peas or mixed veggies to boost the balanced diet. |
| Fruit | Any of your choice. |

Total: zero, again

----

### Dinner
The basic diet is: lean meat/chicken, carbs, veggies and/or fruit.

Sunday is the day most people like to relax, but it's also a big meal day. As with Wednesdays, here is the time for something new or an old favorite revisited with different cooking methods.

Some suggestions include: roasted turkey or chicken, with mashed potatoes, salad, biscuits, and a low-fat cheesecake for dessert; or, a pot roast, with the visible fat taken off before baking with all the trimmings. My favorite is goulash for six, and with five of them frozen for later.

Whatever you decide to do for Sunday, just remember you've worked hard all week, now is not the time to go back to your old ways. ☺

# In closing …

Some may be asking what makes me an expert in diet and nutrition. I'm not, never claimed to be. But reading the guidelines set out by the experts isn't rocket science; it's just simple logic. Coming up with foods that fit those guidelines was a fun challenge; making them tasty and interesting wasn't as difficult as it may seem.

Not every diet is for every one; we're all different. I didn't put in some of my personal preferences as you may or may not like them; so, I've given you a starting point for you to think about which brand you may like better. We all need a place to start; I hope this is yours.

# ~~ **My Menu** ~~

Day: _____

Breakfast: _____

_____

_____

_____

_____

Lunch: _____

_____

_____

_____

Dinner: _____

_____

_____

_____

Snacks: _____

_____

# ~~ My Menu ~~

Day: _____

Breakfast: _____

_____

_____

_____

_____

Lunch: _____

_____

_____

_____

Dinner: _____

_____

_____

_____

Snacks: _____

_____

## ~~ My Menu ~~

Day: _____

Breakfast: _____

_____

_____

_____

_____

Lunch: _____

_____

_____

_____

Dinner: _____

_____

_____

_____

Snacks: _____

_____

## ~~ My Menu ~~

Day: _____

Breakfast: _____

_____

_____

_____

_____

_____

Lunch: _____

_____

_____

_____

Dinner: _____

_____

_____

_____

Snacks: _____

_____

# ~~ My Menu ~~

Day: _____

Breakfast: _____

_____

_____

_____

_____

Lunch: _____

_____

_____

_____

Dinner: _____

_____

_____

_____

Snacks: _____

_____

# ~~ My Menu ~~

Day: _____

Breakfast: _____

_____

_____

_____

_____

Lunch: _____

_____

_____

_____

Dinner: _____

_____

_____

_____

Snacks: _____

_____

# ~~ My Menu ~~

Day: _____

Breakfast: _____

_____

_____

_____

_____

_____

Lunch: _____

_____

_____

_____

Dinner: _____

_____

_____

_____

Snacks: _____

_____

# ~~ My Menu ~~

Day: _____

Breakfast: _____

_____

_____

_____

_____

Lunch: _____

_____

_____

_____

Dinner: _____

_____

_____

_____

Snacks: _____

_____

# ~~ My Menu ~~

Day: _____

Breakfast: _____

_____

_____

_____

_____

Lunch: _____

_____

_____

_____

Dinner: _____

_____

_____

_____

Snacks: _____

_____

# ~~ My Menu ~~

Day: _____

Breakfast: _____

_____

_____

_____

_____

_____

Lunch: _____

_____

_____

_____

Dinner: _____

_____

_____

_____

Snacks: _____

_____

# ~~ My Menu ~~

Day: _____

Breakfast: _____

_____

_____

_____

_____

_____

Lunch: _____

_____

_____

_____

Dinner: _____

_____

_____

_____

Snacks: _____

_____

# ~~ My Menu ~~

Day: _____

Breakfast: _____

_____

_____

_____

_____

Lunch: _____

_____

_____

_____

Dinner: _____

_____

_____

_____

Snacks: _____

_____

# ~~ My Menu ~~

Day: _____

Breakfast: _____

_____

_____

_____

_____

Lunch: _____

_____

_____

_____

Dinner: _____

_____

_____

_____

Snacks: _____

_____

# ~~ My Menu ~~

Day: _____

Breakfast: _____

_____

_____

_____

_____

_____

Lunch: _____

_____

_____

_____

Dinner: _____

_____

_____

_____

_____

Snacks: _____

_____